Plant-Based Diet:

The Simple Plant Base Diet Meal Plan: Beginners Cookbook to Plan Your Meals for Every Week

use or misuse of the information in question by the reader will render any resulting actions solely under their purview.

There are no scenarios in which the publisher or the original author of this work can be in any fashion deemed liable for any hardship or damages that may befall them after undertaking information described herein.

Additionally, the information in the following pages is intended only for informational purposes and should thus be thought of as universal. As befitting its nature, it is presented without assurance regarding its prolonged validity or interim quality. Trademarks that are mentioned are done without written consent and can in no way be considered an endorsement from the trademark holder.

Table of Contents

!Disclaimer!

Before we begin, I would like to point out that this book does not offer professional medical advice. Any Statements within <u>Plant-based Diet</u> are in no way, shape, or form meant to protect or identify certain illnesses. If you have health issues of any kind, please refer to a professional health care specialist. The information provided in this book is meant to be used for educational purpose only and does not claim to be a substitute for doctor or other medical professionals.

Introduction

There are a million and one reasons for someone to start a diet. Before you begin learning about the incredible benefits of the plant-based diet, I invite you to take a few minutes to figure out your why. Why is now the time that you are deciding to change your life? Changing your whole lifestyle can be incredibly overwhelming, but when you want the change bad enough, you will have the mental capacity to overcome any obstacles that stand between you and your goal.

Do you have your why? Excellent. You are most likely here because you have heard about the plant-based diet from social media, friends, or even a family member. The real question you may have is why this diet is any different from the others I have tried? If you have tried other diets and have failed, you are not alone! There was a survey completed in the UK that shows two out of five people will quit their diet in the first seven days! Why do people fail? We are creatures of habit! There are many of us who simply do not like change! For some, this is okay, but if you are seeking true change, you will have to put in some hard work! Will it be easy? Absolutely not! Will it be worth it? By the end of this book, you can be the judge of that!

The plant-based diet is wonderful for a number of different reasons. As you will soon learn, this lifestyle can be easy to follow, is incredibly affordable, and very delicious all at the same time! If it seems too good to be true, pinch yourself because this is the reality of the plant-based diet. While more than likely it is very different from your SAD (Standard American Diet) diet, the change is what people struggle with the most. The good news is that the plant-based diet is meant for individuals who are looking to:

- Lose Weight
- Prevent Disease
- Reverse Disease
- Become Healthier
- Gain Energy
- Save the Planet
- And More!

If any of these reasons appeal to you, the plant-based diet is going to be the way to go! In the chapters to follow, you will be provided with all of the information you need to help you get started! From the benefits to the foods you will be enjoying, I hope that by the end of this book you will be both prepared and excited to get started. The plant-based diet is not a new concept, but with some simple changes to your current lifestyle, you will be reaping the benefits of the diet almost immediately. When you are ready, let's go ahead and get started on your new healthy, plant-based journey!

Chapter One: What is a Plant-based Diet?

Congratulations on making the first step to changing your life for the better! If you have made it to this point, I assume you have decided to give the plant-based diet a flying chance! While many individuals in your life may doubt this lifestyle, you are about to learn that this way of life has helped people since the beginning of time. When you think about it, our ancestors all lived a plant-based diet, and we have made it this far! Unfortunately, we are here, but that doesn't mean we are here and healthy. In fact, there are many sick individuals who begin the plant-based diet to reverse their disease and help with the underlying side effects caused by a bad diet. I invite you to take a step back in history to figure out how we got here in the first place. After all, history is learned, so we never make the same mistakes again!

History of the Plant-based Diet

As you can imagine, humans have been consuming a plant-based diet before we even knew the invention of McDonald's and some of our other favorite fast-food chains. To begin our journey, I am going to start us off in the times of hunter-gatherer. While we could go back even further (think Egypt!), I believe this is where a plant-based diet becomes most relevant!

Hunting and Gathering

During this specific time in human history, the hunter-gatherer time period is where we find the earliest evidence of hunting. While we do have a long history of eating meat, this is a point in time where consuming meat was very limited. Of course, humans eating meat does not mean we were carnivores; in fact, the way we are built tells us differently. Yes, we can consume meat, but humans are considered omnivores more or less. You can tell this by our jaw design, running speeds, alimentary tract, and the fact we don't have claws attached to our fingers. With that being said, history also tells us we are omnivores by nature; however, the evolution of our human brains leads us to become hunters so that we could survive.

The need for hunting did not come around until our ancestors left tropical regions. It was in other locations that started having an effect on the availability of plant-based foods. Instead of enduring winter with limited amounts of food, we had to adapt! Of course, out of hunger, animal-flesh becomes much more appealing. This early in time, our ancestors did not have a grocery store just to pop in and buy whatever they needed. Instead, they used the opportunity of hunting and gathering to keep themselves alive.

Agriculture

Eventually, we moved away from hunting and gathering and started to become farmers! While this timeline is a bit tricky and the agriculture history began at different points in different parts of the world, all that matters is that at some point; animals started to become domesticated and dairy, eggs, and meat all became readily available. Once this started, humans no longer needed to hunt nor gather because the farmers provided everything we could desire!

With that being said, while the harvest of fruits and vegetables could vary depending on the season, animals were always readily available for slaughter or animal-made products. On top of this benefit, animal products added taste to food, variety to the plate, and provided a sufficient amount of fat to help people survive. While humans learned to adapt to eating animal flesh, this doesn't mean that it is better for our health. In fact, you will learn that quite the opposite happened. Through modern science, it was found that as individuals eat more plant-based foods, their risk for disease and obesity decreases.

There are many different examples of a plant-based diet through history along with the vegan and vegetarian lifestyles. As you will be learning in a bit, there are a few differences between the three that will be important for you to understand as you choose this lifestyle. For now, we will go over the basic principles of a plant-based diet so you can decide if this is the best option for you. Once you have figured that out, we can go over the different types of a plant-based diet and the differences between them. Remember that there is no one way to do something right. We are all unique individuals with different goals in mind. At the end of the day, it doesn't matter what your spouse or mother thinks. If you feel something is best for you, go for it!

Basics of a Plant-based Diet

A plant-based diet is so much more than just what you are eating; it is about creating an overall healthier lifestyle. While plant-based diets have a great range depending on your goals, there are some basic principles you will be following no matter which version you decide on.

First off, you will be putting an emphasis on minimally processed foods. This meaning that if your food has a label that includes ingredients you cannot pronounce; it is most likely not allowed on your plant-based diet. Instead of heavily processed foods, you will now be consuming whole foods that will benefit your health instead of causing it to suffer or get worse. On top of this, you will also be limiting or avoiding animal products altogether.

Say goodbye to your chicken nuggets and hello to whole grains, nuts, legumes, fruits, and delicious vegetables! All of these foods will be making up the majority of your diet. In the third chapter, we will be going more in-depth on the foods you will be enjoying and the foods you will be avoiding while on a plant-based diet. You may be surprised to learn how delicious eating plant-based can be! I made sure to include some of my favorite and healthy recipes to help you get started! Unfortunately, there is a common misconception that whole foods are bland in taste. As long as you are using the right spices, that will never be a problem!

On a plant-based diet, you will want to use every opportunity to fuel your body properly. Due to this concept, you will need to learn how to pay more attention to the quality of your food. With that being said, a plant-based diet promotes eating foods that are organic and have been sourced locally whenever possible. While it is a bit more effort, it will be worth it in the long run. All you have to ask yourself is would you rather your money go toward fueling your body in the healthiest way possible or toward a medical bill because you didn't take care of yourself properly in the first place?

Vegan vs. Vegetarian vs. Plant-based

As you can tell from the basic concepts of the plant-based diet, it is often confused with vegan and vegetarian. Granted, there are some similarities; there are also some differences you should be aware of before deciding on any lifestyle. Below, we will go over each lifestyle so you can decide which version is best for you!

Vegetarianism

For most people, becoming a vegetarian is an easy first step. While some individuals become vegetarian for health purposes, others do it for ethical and environmental reasons. Being a vegetarian simply means that you do not consume meat. This means no fish, no pork, no beef, and no chicken. While some people do still consume fish (pescatarians), it should be noted that fish are indeed animals.

The good news is that by simply cutting out meat, individuals experience health benefits from this simple change. When you cut meat from the diet, it is often replaced by grains, vegetables, and fruits. Typically, less meat also means less added sugars and oils as well. This is beneficial as high glycemic index foods increase the risk of obesity, diabetes, and heart disease.

Veganism

Next, we have veganism, which is basically an extreme vegetarian. By becoming a vegan, individuals make the ethical choice to exclude any products that exploit animals for any purpose including clothing and foods. Due to these reasons, vegans have a very strict diet that does not incorporate any animal products. Some of these include honey, eggs, dairy, and even gelatin. There are even some extreme vegans who cut out alcohol due to it being processed through isinglass (bladders of fish) or refined sugars that were processed with bone char.

Much like with vegetarians, veganism has some wonderful health benefits. Vegans eat a wide variety of plant foods including vegetables, fruits, seeds, nuts, grains, and beans. While these are all options, vegans can still consume plant-cheeses, plant-milks, cereal, crackers, and more. You will be surprised to learn what vegans can still consume without feeling alienated from the SAD diet. In fact, many of the fast-food chains we discussed earlier have vegan options!

Plant-based

Finally, we get to the good part! Plant-based is exactly what you think it is! This diet is based all around plants. You can be a vegan and be plant-based. You can be a vegetarian and be plant-based! You can consume a small amount of meat and STILL be plant-based! The point is, the mass majority of your food sources need to come from plants.

While following a plant-based diet, you will want to spend the majority of your days avoiding animal products. When you do choose to consume an animal product, it is suggested you use it as a side dish instead of the main course. Often times, you will see a plant-based diet referred to as a whole food plant-based diet because that is exactly what it is! Your plant-based diet focus is on health and well-being as opposed to ethic or environmental purposes, though you get those benefits out of the diet as well!

The issue with the confusion between plant-based and vegans is that vegans get upset over plant-based individuals calling themselves vegan, especially when they are using non-vegan products and giving vegans a bad rep! Plant-based means you will be eating whole foods. But, what the heck are whole foods? Isn't that a grocery store? Yes; it is a grocery store, but it is also the food you will be eating on a plant-based diet. Basically, this just means you will be eating foods that are in their natural form.

As you can tell, there are some similarities and differences between being vegan, vegetarian, and being plant-based. If you are looking for a diet for ethical reasons, vegan and vegetarian are the way to go. If you are looking for a diet to benefit your health, benefit the animals, and benefit the environment, say hello to a plant-based diet! With that in mind, it is now time to go over the different versions of a plant-based diet. By having the information you need, you can make the choice that best fits your health needs!

Different Plant-based Diets

You may think that starting a plant-based diet is fairly simple (eat plants, done) but there are probably different types of diets that you have never even heard of. In fact, there seem to be just as many plant-based diets are there are non-plant-based diets! Whether you want to focus on cutting certain foods, levels of processed foods, or macronutrient ratio; there is a diet for just about every person out there! The one thing that can be agreed on is that plant-based foods are best for health purposes! The best part is that each diet has the ability or be tweaked and changed to fit anyone's lifestyle. As you learn about each version, feel free to take the concepts and make them your own to fit your specific lifestyle.

As you will soon find out, there are advantages and disadvantages of each plant-based diet. Before we continue, I invite you to remember your why again. Are you here to lose weight? Reverse disease? Prevent disease in the first place? I want you to keep your why in mind as we move forward and remember that you need to choose which is best for you and forget what anyone else thinks of it!

Whole Food Plant Based

If you are a beginner with a plant-based diet, this is typically an excellent place to start. This diet is all about eating plants exclusively. This means that you will be consuming foods that are as unprocessed as possible. With that being said, you will never need to count a calorie or pay attention to your macronutrients while following a plant-based diet. With plants being a majority of your diet, you will find that these foods contain fiber and are very nutrient dense; this meaning you will fill up before you even have the chance of consuming too many calories!

Focused Foods:

- Raw and Cooked Vegetables
- Nuts and Seeds
- Whole Fruits
- ALL the legumes
- Unprocessed Whole Grains

The Starch Solution

If you are like me, your eyes probably got wide at the thought of consuming more starch. This plant-based diet is a very successful program started by Dr. John McDougall. This diet is starch-based along with healthy portions of vegetables and fruits. McDougall's focus was around how older generations thrived off of a starch-based diet while their children and grandchildren became sicker and fatter of animal products. If you have health issues that you believe is being caused by your diet (think oils and animal products) this program is based around fueling the body properly to help the body thrive and heal itself.

Focused Foods:

- Potatoes
- Starches (Millet, Quinoa, Barley, Wheat, Rice, Corn)
- Vegetables (Non-starchy and Starchy)
- Fruits (Limited Servings-3 Per Day)
- Nuts and Seeds (Discouraged or Limited)

Nutritarian

This is also known as the "eat to live," diet invented by Dr. Joel Fuhrman. Fuhrman wanted to create a diet that was both optimal for humans and nutrient dense. While on this diet it is recommended to eat a mass majority of vegetables, animal products are added in after a few weeks of following the nutritarian diet strictly. Unlike with the starch solution, it is limited on this diet. If you have a weak digestive system, this will not be the best option for you. One of the major concepts of this diet is G.B.O.M.B.S. This meaning that individuals on this diet will be eating greens, beans, onions, mushrooms, multiple types of berries and seeds. If you are looking to slim down, this diet is oil-free and low in salt and could benefit you greatly.

Focused Foods:

- Nuts and Seeds

- Mushrooms
- Onions and Garlic
- Fresh Fruit
- Green Vegetables
- Beans

Low Fat Raw Vegan Diet

More than likely, you have heard of this version of a whole food, plant-based diet. It is typically referred to as the 80/10/10 diet where individuals are asked to focus on eating fresh organic fruits that are ripe and whole along with seeds, nuts, and some leafy greens. The popularity of this diet took off by YouTubers who were passionate vegans. If you live in a warmer climate, this may be the perfect plant-based diet for you as you will most likely have a bigger selection of ripe fruit at any given time.

Focused Foods:

- Raw Seeds and Nuts
- Green Leafy Veggies
- Savory Fruits
- All Types of Fresh Fruits

SOS-Free Diet

Another popular plant-based diet would be the SOS-free diet. In this case, SOS stands for sugar, oil, and salt. If you struggle with binge eating or overeating, this could be the perfect option for you! This is a plant-based diet which eliminates three major stimulants to your average diet. When we have salt and sugar added to our foods, it makes it easier to eat because they are that much more palatable. These three stimulants referred to as "The Pleasure Trap," shows that people enjoy getting pleasure without having to work hard for it. Eventually, this can lead to addiction for some people. While it may seem a bit extreme, it is a good choice for those who typically overindulge with their meals.

Focused Foods:

- Beans and Lentils
- Whole Grains
- Vegetables
- Fruits
- Small Portions of Seeds and Nuts

Whole Starch Low Fat

This is much like the starch solution version of a plant-based diet with a few different tweaks. If you are looking to lose weight while following a plant-based diet, this could be the perfect option for you! This version of the diet is high carbohydrate but low fat. The issue many people seem to have on a plant-based diet is replacing meats with processed junk foods. Instead, individuals on a whole starch, low-fat diet are asked to fill up on starches for all of their meals. While following this, refined foods and oils are cut out, and salt and simple sugars are limited. Typically, this way of eating is to be followed through the week and becomes much more relaxed on the weekend. This type of plant-based diet is attractive to vegans who came from a more restrictive version of the diet.

Focused Foods:

- Vegetables
- Fruit for Breakfast
- Legumes
- Potatoes
- Brown Rice
- Corn
- Quinoa
- Pumpkin

Engine 2 Diet

While I could go on and on about the different, wonderful versions of the plant-based diet, we will end this chapter on the engine 2 Diet. If you are looking to lose weight and improve your overall health, this will be the plant-based diet for you. By following this specific program, individuals were able to lose weight, lower their cholesterol, and become very healthy versions of themselves. The main focus here is on plant-based foods and keeping fat intake low. All oils and animal products are excluded on the Engine 2 Diet, but refined sugars and sodium are allowed in very limited portions.

Focused Foods:

- Nuts and Seeds
- Nut Butters
- Fruits and Dried Fruits
- Green Vegetables
- Legumes
- Whole Grains

At this point, your head must be spinning! Starting a plant-based diet can seem overwhelming at first, but I promise with the right information provided, you will be ready to start in no time! If you are like me, it is probably confusing to start this way of life as we have been taught all of our life about the "vital role" animal products have in our life and diet. More than likely, you are wondering how you are going to replace these nutrients that you usually receive from dairy, eggs, and meat.

Right now, I don't want you to worry about that! As you begin your new lifestyle, there is no need to stress over changing everything in a day. Each and every meal, you will have the decision to choose which foods are best for you. Are you going to slip up? Absolutely! Is that okay? Yes! The main point is that you are now making the conscious decision to better your health. Over time and with practice, you will learn how to balance your lifestyle to your liking.

In the next chapter, we will begin to go over the incredible benefits a plant-based diet can bring into your life. Whether you are doing this for weight loss, health benefits, lifestyle benefits, or for the environmental impact; prepare to be convinced to start a plant-based diet today. I hope you are ready to better your life because that is exactly what will happen when you begin to fuel your body properly!

Chapter Two: Benefits of a Plant-Based Diet

While starting a plant-based diet is an excellent idea and has many wonderful benefits let's be honest, you are mostly here to benefit yourself. I am not here to judge! It is fantastic that you are deciding to put you and your health first! You deserve to be the best version of yourself, with a little bit of legwork, you will be there in no time!

To some people, a plant-based diet is just another fad diet. There are so many diets on the market right now, why is plant-based any different? Whether you are looking to lose weight, reverse disease, or just love animals; the plant-based diet can help you out in a number of different ways! On this diet, you will become healthy on the inside and healthy on the outside.

A plant-based diet is so much more than just eating fruits and vegetables. This is a lifestyle where you are encouraged to journey to a better version of yourself. As you improve your eating habits, you will need something to do with all of your new found energy! It is time to gain control over your eating habits and figure out how food truly does affect our daily lives! Below, you will find the amazing benefits a plant-based diet has to offer you.

Reason Number One: Lower Your Cholesterol

Let me start by asking you a question; how much do you think one egg affects your cholesterol? One egg a day could increase your dietary cholesterol from 97 to 418 mg in a single day! There was a study done on seventeen lacto-vegetarian college students. During this <u>study,</u> the students were asked to consume 400kcal in test foods along with one large egg for three weeks. During this time, their dietary cholesterol raised to these numbers. To put it in perspective, 200 to 239 mg/dL is considered borderline high.

The next question you should be asking yourself is what is considered a healthy amount of cholesterol? The answer is zero percent! There is no tolerable intake of trans fats, saturated fats, nor cholesterol. All of these (found in animal products) raise LDL cholesterol. Luckily, a plant-based diet can bring your cholesterol levels down drastically. By doing this, you will be lowering your risk of disease that is typically related to high cholesterol levels. The good news here is that your body makes the cholesterol you need! There is no need to "get it" from other sources.

Reason Number Two: Healthy Antioxidants

As of recently, there has been a push with products showing they are incredibly healthy due to the fact they contain antioxidants. These are fantastic as antioxidants help prevent the circulation of oxidized fats that are building up in your bloodstream. As you consume more antioxidants naturally in your plant-based diet, this can help reduce inflammation, lower your blood pressure, prevent blood clots, and decrease any artery stiffness you may have.

To put it into perspective, a plant can contain about sixty-four times more antioxidants compared to animal products such as meat. In the chapter to follow, you will be learning more about the foods that contain antioxidants and how to incorporate them into your diet. The good news is that these foods are healthy, natural, and delicious all at the same time!

Reason Number Three: High Fiber Intake

As you begin a plant-based diet, you will be getting more fiber in your diet naturally. You may be surprised to learn that on average, about ninety percent of Americans do not receive the proper amount of fiber! This is bad news for a majority of people as fiber has some very good benefits. Fiber has been shown to reduce the <u>risk</u> of stroke, obesity, heart disease, diabetes, breast cancer, and the <u>risk</u> of colon cancer! On top of these benefits, fiber also helps control blood sugar levels and cholesterol levels.

Reason Number Four: Asthma Benefits

According to the Centers for Disease Control and Prevention, about ten percent of children in 2009 has asthma. This means that in 2009, more children than adults had the risk of having an asthma attack. Asthma is defined as an inflammatory disease. The question is, what is causing the rise of asthma? You guessed it; it's all in the diet! According to one study, both eggs and sweetened beverages have been linked to asthma. On the other hand, fruits and vegetables both appear to have a positive effect on lowering asthma in children that eat at least two servings of vegetables a day. In fact, their risk of suffering from an allergic asthma attack was lowered by fifty percent!

Reason Number Five: Reduce Risk of Breast Cancer

While it can be hard to pinpoint the development of breast cancer, it seems there are three steps to creating a healthier lifestyle to lower your risk of developing it in the first place. First, you will want to maintain a normal body weight. Luckily, this can be achieved by consuming a plant-based diet. On top of eating your fruits and vegetables, you will also want to limit your alcohol consumption. By doing this, individuals have been able to reduce <u>their risk</u> of developing breast cancer by sixty percent! To put this into perspective, meat eaters have a seventy-four percent higher <u>risk</u> of developing breast cancer compared to those who eat more vegetables. I'm not sure about you, but that just doesn't seem worth it to me!

Reason Number Six: Reduce the Development of Kidney Stones

Did you know that by eating one extra can of tuna a day can increase your <u>risk</u> of forming a calcium stone in your urinary tract by a whopping two-hundred and fifty percent? The risk is calculated by studying the relative probability of forming a stone when high animal protein is ingested. The theory behind this is that urine needs to be more alkaline if you want to lower your risk of developing stones. When meat is consumed, this produced acid in the body. On the other hand, beans and vegetables both reduce the acid in the body, leading to a lower risk of developing kidney stones; science!

Reason Number Seven: Reverse and Prevent High Blood Pressure and Heart Disease

Unfortunately, one in three Americans has high blood pressure. Studies have shown that as a diet becomes plant-based, this grants the ability to drop the rate of hypertension. In fact, there is about a <u>seventy-five</u> percent drop between an omnivore and a vegan! It appears as though a vegetarian diet sets a kind of protection against cardiometabolic risk factors, cardiovascular disease, as well as overall total mortality. When compared against a lacto-ovo-vegetarian diet, plant-based diets seem to also have protection against cardiovascular mortality, type-2 diabetes, hypertension, as well as obesity! This is fantastic news, especially when you lean that just three portions of whole-grain foods seem to significantly reduce the <u>risk</u> of cardiovascular disease in middle-aged people. This is the same benefit that a symptom-reducing drug can give you!

Reason Number Eight: Control and Prevent Cancer

To start this little section off, I will inform you that fat from animals is often associated with the <u>risk</u> of developing pancreatic cancer. In fact, for every fifty grams of chicken consumed on a daily basis, your risk of developing pancreatic cancer increases by seventy-two percent! At this point in time, pancreatic cancer is the fourth most common death-causing cancer in the world. It's pretty simple to avoid if you simply switch your beef to beans!

On the other end of the spectrum, it appears that by consuming 70g of more beans a day can cut your <u>risk</u> of developing colon cancer by seventy-five percent. This may be due to IP (6) which is found in cereal and beans. It appears this plays a major role in controlling tumor-growth, metastasis and preventing cancer. In addition to these benefits, IP (6) overall seems to enhance the immune system, lower elevated serum cholesterol, prevent calcification and kidney stones, as well as reducing pathological platelet activity within the body. That seems pretty nifty for eating just a few more beans and less meat!

Reason Number Nine: Decrease Insulin Resistance

Our bodies are very delicate machines. When fat begins to accumulate in your muscle cells, this interferes with insulin. When this build up happens, the insulin in the body is unable to bring the sugar out of the blood system that your body needs for energy. Unfortunately, high sugar intake makes this situation even worse and can clog your arteries altogether. When you eliminate meat from the diet, this means you will have less fat in your muscles. By decreasing these levels, you will be able to avoid insulin resistance in the first place!

Reason Number Ten: Reverse and Prevent Diabetes

I am going to start off with the bad news. As of right now, diabetes is the cause of 750,000 deaths each year. Since 1990, the number of individuals in the United States diagnosed with diabetes has tripled to more than twenty million people. Within this range, you have one-hundred and thirty-two thousand children below the age of eighteen years old who suffer from diabetes. In 2014, fifty-two thousand people were diagnosed with end-age renal disease due to diabetes. Overall, the United States spent a total of two hundred and forty-five billion dollars in direct cost of diagnosing individuals with diabetes. If these numbers seem overwhelming to you, I have good news; plant-based diet can help with this issue. As you learn how to incorporate more vegetables into your diet, the risk of developing hypertension and diabetes drops by about seventy-eight percent.

Reason Number Eleven: Obesity Control and Weight Loss

In a study completed on various diet groups, it was shown that beans typically have a lower mass index compared to other individuals. These people were also proven to be less prone to obesity when they were compared to both vegetarians and non-vegetarians. This may be due to the fact that plant-based individuals have lower animal intake and higher fiber intake. When you reduce your caloric intake to lose weight at an unhealthy level, this has the ability to lead to unhealthy coping mechanisms such as bulimia and anorexia. As you learn how to follow a plant-based diet, you will be filling up on healthy foods such as vegetables, fruits, nuts, and whole grains. At no point on this diet should you be starving or wishing you could eat more. All of the food you will be consuming are typically low in fat and will help with weight loss.

Reason Number Twelve: Healthier Bones

One of the common misconceptions around a plant-based diet is that due to the fact you will no longer be drinking cow's milk, you will be lacking the calcium your bones need to grow strong. While we will be going over this further in depth later, all you need to know now is that it simply is not true. While on a plant-based diet, you will be receiving plenty of essential nutrients such as vitamin K, magnesium, and potassium; all of which improve bone health.

A plant-based diet helps maintain an acid-base ratio which is very important for bone health. While on an acidic diet, this aids in the loss of calcium during urination. As you learned earlier, the more meat you consume, the more acidic your body becomes. Luckily, fruits and vegetables are high in magnesium and potassium which provides alkalinity in your diet. This means that through diet, you will be able to reduce the bone resorption.

Along the same lines, green leafy vegetables are filled with vitamin K that you need for your bones. Studies have shown that with an adequate amount of vitamin K in your diet, this can help reduce the risk of hip fractures. Along with these studies, research has also shown that soy products that have isoflavones also have a positive effect on bone health in women that are postmenopausal. By having a proper amount of isoflavones, this helps improve bone mineral density, reduce bone resorption, and helps improve overall bone formation. Overall, less calcium loss leads to reducing your risk of osteoporosis, even when calcium intake is low!

Reason Number Thirteen: Do it for the Animals

Whether or not you are switching to a plant-based diet for reasons other than health, it never hurts to be kind and compassionate toward other sentient beings. At the end of the day, sparing someone's life is going to be the right thing to do, especially when they never asked to be brought into this world in the first place. Unfortunately, this is the whole reason behind the dairy and meat industry. In all honesty, there is nothing humane about taking lives or animal farming.

Of course, this goes beyond meat products. There are also major issues with the egg and dairy industry where dairy cows are forcefully impregnated and then have their calves taken away so we can steal their milk. These animals have feelings and emotions just like we do, what gives us the right to use them for their worth and then throw them away like garbage when we no longer have a use for them? Do the animals a favor and eat more plants, it will be better on your conscious.

Along with these same lines, you never know what is going to come with your animal products. There are a host of toxins, dioxins, hormones, antibiotics, and bacteria that can cause some serious health issues. In fact, there is a very high percentage of animal flesh that is contaminated with dangerous bacteria such as E. coli, listeria, and Campylobacter. These are all tough to find some time because these bacteria live in the flesh, feces, and intestinal tracts of the animals.

With the bacteria being tough to find and kill, this eventually can cause food poisoning. Each year, the USDA has reported that animal flesh causes about seventy percent of food poisoning per year. This means that there are about seventy-five million cases of food poisoning a year, five-thousands of which result in death.

Reason Number Fourteen: Do it for the Environment

We were given this one planet to live on, and we should be doing everything in our power to help protect it. During these trying times, it seems that half of the population believes in climate change while the other half thinks of it as fake news. As a plant-eater, it is our duty to do our part in saving the environment. Unfortunately, the meat and farming industry is going to be a hard beast to take down. Depending on the source, it has been proven that the meat industry is behind anywhere from eighteen to fifty-one percent of man-made pollution. This puts the farm industry ahead of transportation when it comes down to the contribution of pollution to the greenhouse effect. In one pound of hamburger meat that you are consuming, this equals about seventy-five kg of CO_2 emission. Do you know what produces that much CO_2 emission? Three weeks from using your car! Do your part, eat more plants and save the planet.

Reason Number Fifteen: Improve your Mood

When you are making an impact on saving the animals and saving the environment, it is no surprise that your mood will enhance! As you begin to cut back on animal products, you will be abstaining from the stress hormones those animals are producing while they are on their way to the slaughterhouse. This factor alone will have a major <u>impact</u> on your mood stability. By eating plants, this helps individuals lower their levels of fatigue, hostility, anger, depression, anxiety, and overall tension. The mood boost may be due to the antioxidants mentioned earlier in this chapter.

On top of these added benefits, it seems as though carbohydrate-rich foods like rye bread, steel cut oats, and brown rice all seem to have a positive effect on the serotonin levels in the brain. Serotonin is very important in controlling mood which is why a plant-based diet may help treat the symptoms that are often associated with depression and anxiety.

Reason Number Sixteen: Skin and Digestion Improvements

You may be surprised to learn that skin and digestion are actually connected! If you suffer from acne-prone skin, dairy may be the culprit behind the issue! If you have bad acne, try a plant-based diet. As you eat more fruits and vegetables, you will be eliminating fatty foods such as oils and animal products that may be causing the acne in the first place. On top of this, fruits and vegetables are often rich in water and can provide you with high levels of minerals and vitamins. By consuming more fiber in your diet, this helps eliminate toxins in your body and boost digestion. When this happens, it could clear up your acne!

Reason Number Seventeen: Improve Overall Fitness

Amazing things will happen as you lose weight and clean yourself from the inside out. When people first begin a plant-based diet, there is a common misconception that a lack of animal products means a lack of muscle mass and energy. Luckily, the opposite is true. It seems as though meat and dairy are both harder to digest. When these products are harder to digest, this means that it is taking more energy to do so. As you consume more fruits and vegetables on a plant-based diet, you will be amazed at how much added energy and strength you will develop.

On top of these benefits, a plant-based diet provides you with plenty of great quality proteins if you are looking to build muscle mass. While eating legumes, nuts, seeds, green vegetables, and whole grains, you will easily be consuming the forty to fifty grams of protein per day that is recommended. Of course, this number will vary but depending on your goals; you will easily be able to consume plenty of protein on a plant-based diet.

Reason Number Eighteen: It's So Easy

When you first begin a plant-based diet, you should just expect your friends and family to doubt your life choices. You will be amazed to learn just how easy it is to live plant-based in the modern age. At the grocery store alone, there are incredible plant-based options for you and your family. There are plenty of plant-based milk options, ice creams, mock meats and more. In fact, the alternative sales in the market are expected to each about five billion dollars by 2020! Along with supermarkets, more restaurants are choosing to provide plant-based options as well. Now, you are no longer forced to cook at home if you wish to live this lifestyle. With each passing day, becoming a plant-based person is become much easier compared to earlier times.

Along with it becoming easier, it is also an economical choice. As you narrow your food choices down to seasonal fruits, vegetables, seeds, nuts, beans, and grains, you may be surprised to learn how much you will be cutting down your monthly food expenses! One of the best parts of whole foods is that you can buy them in bulk! When you purchase your foods this way, you will be spending less in a day and less on eating out. Luckily, there are plenty of options for eating plant-based on a diet. We will be going more in depth later in the book, be sure to stick around!

Possible Vegan Side Effects

Much like with any choices we make in our lives; there are always going to be benefits and downfalls. I don't want you to jump into a plant-based lifestyle thinking that everything is going to be perfect and dandy. While yes, there are some amazing benefits that come along with fueling your body properly, there is always the risk of possible side effects. Below, we will go over some of the side effects you should be watching out for.

Side Effect Number One: Energy Issues

As you begin your new diet and begin eating more plant-based, without even realizing it, you will be consuming fewer calories! This is due to the fact that most plants have a lower calorie density compared to the foods that are derived from animals. For most people, this means that you will have to eat more food in order for you to receive the calories your body needs to function. For some, this is awesome! For others, this can be a very difficult task at hand.

Unfortunately, undereating will put you at risk of some health issues. In order to avoid this issue, you may want to track your food intake for a couple of days when you first get started. You may feel like you are eating a lot of food, but often times the calories just won't add up the same. Luckily, these foods will be providing the proper antioxidants, minerals, and vitamins you need to energize yourself so you will not be lacking in that department!

Along the same lines, individuals have claimed that when they switch to a plant-based diet, they feel very sluggish. If you begin to feel this way, it could mean that you are either undereating or you are not eating the proper foods to fuel yourself efficiently. Remember that there is a lot of plant-based junk food. While yes, these are within the diet restrictions, this does not mean that they are any better for you than fries and a burger from your favorite fast food joint.

So, what is the game plan if you feel you are losing energy when you switch to a plant-based diet? You will need to take a good, hard look at the foods you are putting into your body. I want you to make sure that the foods you are choosing are whole. These foods will need to be eaten at a higher volume in order to obtain the nutrition and energy you need. As you do this, be sure to avoid all oils and processed sugars. If you complete this, you should have much more energy and feel better than before!

Side Effect Number Two: Cravings

Changing your dietary habits is not going to be an easy task. Unfortunately, we are typically habitual creatures; this meaning that our bodies like the routine of what we do and what we like. Our taste buds are the same exact way! As you change your diet to more vegetables and fruits, you should expect to have cravings for non-plant-based foods. This is especially true if you are not eating enough (see side effect number one) or your body simply wants a certain calorically dense food.

One of the best ways to overcome cravings is to not get wild and crazy with your diet change if you are just getting started. Instead of cutting everything cold turkey, take reasonable steps to remove your favorite foods from your diet. As you do this, you will want to find foods to replace these favorites with. Luckily, there are plenty of healthy and delicious alternatives to help get you past your cravings. Do you want something sweet? Try coconut ice cream or even rice milk chocolate! As you begin to distance yourself from unhealthy, processed foods, I promise you will begin to crave them less!

To help overcome cravings, I suggest you set yourself up for success! The first step will be to remove all temptation from your home. This way, when you reach for your old habits, they won't be at your disposal. Once this is complete, find plant-based versions of your favorite foods. Eventually, your taste buds will adjust to your new way of life, and you may be surprised what healthy foods you will begin to crave!

Side Effect Number Three: Digestive Issues

More than likely, you saw this coming the moment you read that a big part of this diet is beans; we all know the poem about beans! As you begin a plant-based diet, you may begin to experience an uncomfortable feeling in your stomach after your meals. I want to go ahead and say now that you cannot blame the food! Our bodies adjust to food depending on what we eat, and the bacteria found in our gut will optimize itself to digest whatever it needs whether we are eating processed junk or healthy whole foods.

As you begin to change the composition of food from animal products to vegetables, legumes, and grains, you may be changing slightly too sudden for your body. Unfortunately, this has the potential to lead to bloating, diarrhea, or even constipation. Why you ask? Fiber.

Fiber is an indigestible part of plants that for the most part, are not typically found in processed foods nor animal products. However; fiber is crucial for the body's ability to digest food properly and our overall health. In fact, fiber is the reason we are able to move the junk of our food out, so we become, ahem, regular.

Along with becoming more regular, fiber also will help you lower your risk for chronic disease and aids the body in nutrient absorption. Yes, you will be using the bathroom more, but this is actually a really good thing. Eventually, your body will transition to the new food and will get over the digestive distress. As your digestion becomes smoother, you will no longer have stomach pains, and you will actually begin to feel lighter!

Side Effect Number Four: Social Struggles

As mentioned earlier, many people will doubt your new diet choice. We happen to live in a very carnist society where many of our meals revolve around meat. Think about this for a second; what do you typically eat at a baseball game? Hamburgers and Hot Dogs? You go out to your favorite restaurant; what do you typically order? More than likely, this meal revolves around meat with the vegetable on the side! As you switch over the more plants, set yourself up for success by expecting a backlash.

When people first start off with a plant-based diet, this can be a true test for individuals. You may be shocked to learn how many of your friends are suddenly "nutritionist" and will tell you about everything you are missing out on by not consuming animal flesh. While it may be hard to hear, I suggest you never allow anyone to keep you from living your life the way you want.

While it may be difficult to go out with friends now, that does not mean that it is impossible. As mentioned earlier, the world is becoming more plant-friendly as we continue to evolve and change the meaning of what it is to be plant-based. At the end of the day, it does not matter what anyone says to you or what they think of your life choices. You are very well aware of the incredible benefits this diet has to offer you, and that is all that matters! Instead of fighting back when the small comments come, simply prepare yourself and be ready to answer all stupid and legit questions that revolve around a plant-based diet. Those who truly care for you will understand.

Potential Nutritional Shortfalls

When you begin a plant-based diet, you will need to be mindful about your essential nutrients. On a plant-based diet, there are a few potential nutritional shortfalls if you are not careful about what you are eating on a daily basis. Some of these missing vitamins and minerals will be essential if you wish to continue a proper body function. Below, we will go over some of the more popular shortfalls plant-based individuals run into. The hope is that by being mindful from the beginning, you can avoid the issue in the first place.

Vitamin B12

If you become deficient in vitamin B12, you enter the risk of bone breakage, elevated levels of homocysteine, abnormal neurological symptoms and anemia. B12 can be found in a number of different foods such as nutritional yeast, seaweed, B12 fortified foods, and soy drinks. As we age, the absorption of vitamin B12 begins to deteriorate. Due to this fact, it is normally advised to take a vitamin B12 supplement.

Vitamin D

In general, a plant-based diet has been known to low in vitamin D. When you are low in vitamin D; this could mess with the absorption of calcium in your body. As a result, this could potentially lead to brittle bones. It is suggested you expose yourself to a proper amount of sunlight or consider taking a supplement to help meet your requirements. On top of this, you can also consume foods such as juice, rice milk and soy beverages that have been fortified with vitamin D.

Calcium

As mentioned earlier, calcium is going to be a shortcoming while on a plant-based diet, especially if you typically get your calcium from cow's milk. Instead, you will want to begin consuming dark green leafy vegetables to get your calcium in. Other food sources would include calcium-fortified breakfast cereals, soy beverages, and even calcium. This will help grow strong bones and keep you healthy overall.

Iron

Iron is another supplement that will be vital on your plant-based diet. This is very important for the formation of red blood cells within your body. In order to avoid deficiency of iron, you can consume iron-fortified foods like dry fruits and dark green vegetables. It should be noted that plant-based iron is typically less absorbable by the body compared to those on a meat-based diet. While not impossible, it is harder.

Protein

Protein is a big factor that we will be going over later in this book. There are many individuals who feel it is impossible to get a proper amount of protein on a plant-based diet, but it simply is not true. There is no need to consume eggs, dairy products, and meat to get the proper amount of protein. You can find protein in nuts, seeds, legumes, whole grains, and other vegetable proteins.

Zinc

Finally, we have zinc. Zinc is important in the diet as it helps build a healthy immune system. As you switch over to a plant-based diet, it should be noted that you will have higher concentrations of phytates in your body, making the absorption of dietary minerals slower compared to a meat-based diet. This can be helped by eating zinc-rich foods like legumes, nuts, whole grains, and even pumpkin seeds.

There are a number of different reasons you should make the dive and switch to a plant-based diet. While there are downfalls, you can see that there is always a solution. I am not saying that a plant-based diet is meant for everyone, but it certainly doesn't hurt to try! After all, you are just eating healthier, and it doesn't hurt that you are helping animals and the environment along the way.

I hope that at this point, you are convinced to make the switch to becoming a healthier version of you. In the next chapter, it is time to go over the delicious foods you will be able to consume on a plant-based diet along with the foods you should begin to limit. Once you have a grasp on these foods, I will also be providing you with some of my favorite plant-based recipes along with a grocery list to make it even easier! Be prepared to be mind-blown on just how delicious eating plant-based can truly be.

Chapter Three: Foods to Avoid and Enjoy

Now we get to the good part; eating! To start this chapter off, I first want to go over all of the food you will be able to enjoy while following a plant-based diet. There is a tremendous amount of people who like to focus on the bad when they start a diet, which is exactly why a mass majority of diets fail in the first place! Instead of focusing on what you will no longer be "allowed" to eat on your diet, it is time to learn all of the incredible foods you will be able to enjoy!

Grains

As we go through this section, I want you to imagine the food pyramid we grew up learning in school. At the very bottom of the pyramid, you will find grains; meaning that these are going to be a majority of your new diet. In fact, the recommended daily serving is about six servings of half of a cup of grains per day. As you choose grains, you will want to place a heavy emphasize on whole grains such as buckwheat, wheat berries, millet, quinoa, and brown rice.

There are other choices such as pasta, bread, and cereal but you will want to assure that these selections are as unprocessed as possible. In fact, a mass majority of your calories should come from whole starches. You will be able to consume these foods until you are satiated! As you practice a plant-based diet, you will learn how to adjust your daily servings according to your own energy needs.

Luckily, starches are both healthy and reliable while following a plant-based diet These foods will contain a large number of complex carbohydrates which means you will stay full while getting long-lasting energy to both your brain and your body! On top of these incredible benefits, starches also provide you with minerals, fibers, essential fats, and proteins you need to improve overall health.

Whole Grains Examples

- Wild Rice
- Whole Grain Pasta/ Flour/ Rolls
- Wheat
- Spelt
- Rye
- Quinoa
- Millet
- Farro
- Corn
- Buckwheat
- Brown Rice
- Barley
- Amaranth

Vegetables

The next tier up on the food pyramid for a plant-based diet is going to be vegetables. More than likely, you probably expected this one! For a daily recommendation, you should be striving for five or more servings of either half a cup cooked or one cup raw. In the beginning, this may seem like a difficult task, but with some extra work, every meal will include a vegetable. As you choose your vegetables, imagine that you are trying to eat the rainbow! You will be filling your plate with leafy greens and starchy root vegetables.

As you include more vegetables in your diet, you may find it difficult to eat the large bulk of the food. Remember that on a plant-based diet, it is going to be vital you receive enough calories so you can keep your energy levels up. To solve this "problem," you can always try to consume more soups and smoothies so you can receive the proper amount of nutrients. From this point on, vegetables are going to be your new best friend!

The best part about vegetables is that they are absolute nutrient powerhouses. Vegetables are filled with the phytonutrients, antioxidants, vitamins, minerals, and fiber that your body needs in order to thrive. Whether you are eating these vegetables frozen, fresh, cooked, or raw; there are plenty of options for you to try out on a plant-based diet!

Fresh Vegetable Examples:

- Zucchini
- Yams

- Tomatoes
- Sweet Potato
- Squash
- Pumpkin
- Onion
- Mushrooms
- Green Onions
- Celery
- Cauliflower
- Carrots
- Broccoli
- Bell Peppers
- Asparagus
- Avocado

Leafy Green Examples:

- Wheatgrass
- Spring Greens
- Lettuce
- Kale
- Bok Choy
- Baby Spinach
- Arugula

Fruits

Next, we have the fruit tier. Generally, you will want to eat a lower number of servings of fruits as they are generally higher in natural sugars. If you are looking to lose weight on a plant-based diet, try keeping fruit to about four servings of fruit at half of a cup per day. This way, you keep your fruit consumption in moderation. On a plant-based diet, you can choose fresh fruit, but dried food can be consumed in smaller portions. As a general note, you will want to try to avoid or limit fruit juices.

Luckily, there is a wide variety of fruits for you to choose from and you can still have them on a daily basis. Many fruits are packed with phytonutrients, antioxidants, enzymes, minerals, and the vitamins you need in order to prevent disease and feel healthier. The simple sugars in these fruits are excellent for quick energy if you want to have them as a snack.

As a general rule, you will want to consume fruit that is ripe. At this point, the fruit is both alkalizing and as nutritious as they are going to get. Fruit is wonderful and versatile as you can have them in smoothies, on your oatmeal, or all by itself. Just remember that for the best health benefits on a plant-based diet, you will still need to enjoy "nature's candy" in moderation.

Fresh Fruit Examples:

- Watermelon
- Strawberries
- Raspberries
- Plums
- Peaches
- Oranges

- Mangos
- Limes
- Lemons
- Cucumber
- Blueberries
- Bananas
- Apricots

Legumes

This category will change depending on the version of the plant-based diet you choose to follow. Some dietitians say you should be eating more legumes while others say it should be limited. Cooked beans and lentils are both excellent choices and should be calcium-fortified whenever possible. This is where you are going to get a majority of your protein from. As a general rule, strive for three, half cup servings per day. Below, you will find some of the more popular versions to get you started!

Legume Examples:

- White Beans
- Split Peas
- Snow Peas
- Red Beans
- Pinto Beas
- Lentils
- Kidney Beans
- Green Beans

- Chickpeas
- Black Beans
- Bean Sprouts

Nuts and Seeds

Finally, we reach the top of your plant-based food pyramid! All the way up here, you will find your nuts and seeds. Being such a small portion of the pyramid, you will want to make sure that you keep these to a minimum at one-ounce servings, twice a day. This rule will need to be stricter for those of you who are looking to lose weight while following a plant-based diet.

Individuals who follow a SAD diet receive much more than the recommended 30% calories from fat; all of which are provided from saturated fats and trans fats. For this reason alone, fat generally has a terrible reputation. The truth of the matter is that unprocessed fats you receive from whole foods are healthy and help support a number of functions within the body. In fact, fats are needed to develop a properly functioning brain and nervous systems! Fat is what helps absorb vitamins and minerals into our body to ensure cell health.

Of course, everything needs to be enjoyed in moderation. There is no reason to go overboard with the fats even though it is very easy to do. It is suggested you enjoy a wide variety of healthy plant fats, so you consume the proper number of Omega-3 and Omega-6 Fatty Acids. Below, you will find some of the healthier versions to include in your diet as you go more plant-based.

Nut Examples:

- Walnuts
- Pine Nuts
- Macadamia Nuts
- Hazelnuts
- Cashews
- Almonds

Seed Examples:

- Sunflower Seeds
- Pumpkin Seeds
- Hemp Seeds
- Flax Seeds
- Chia Seeds

Critical Nutritional Needs

When you begin a plant-based diet, it will be vital that you pay special attention to the critical nutrients you need. I don't want you to look at this as a downfall because it certainly will be no issue when you are eating the proper foods, but it may be something you need to focus on when you first start. Below, we will go over some of the popular nutrients you will need and how to receive them through a plant-based diet!

Calcium

For most adults, the daily recommended intake of calcium should be about one thousand milligrams. For elderly people and teenagers, this number will be slightly more. Calcium is very important as it is needed for both nerve and muscle function. As you increase your calcium intake, you will also need an adequate amount of vitamin D in order to properly absorb the calcium into your system. Luckily, there are plenty of soy products that are fortified with calcium!

Foods Examples:

- Almonds
- Tahini
- Soy Milk
- Calcium Tofu
- White Beans
- Navel Oranges
- Kale
- Broccoli
- Spinach
- Collard Greens

Iron

Next, iron will be a vital part of your plant-based diet. For females, the recommended amount per day is about eighteen milligrams; for females, it is only eight. Females typically need more iron during their reproductive years due to monthly blood loss. This iron is necessary for any given diet as it is in charge of transporting oxygen through the body. Iron is also beneficial for DNA synthesis and overall immune system support.

It should be noted that the iron that comes from plant sources are non-home iron, which typically isn't as well absorbed compared to the animal product iron known as home iron. What we do know is that iron from plants is safer to consume compared to the type that comes from animal products. As you increase your iron levels, you will want to add more vitamin C to enhance iron absorption. It is also beneficial to decrease coffee or tea consumption after meals, which messes with the absorption cycle.

Food Examples:

- Green Peas
- Chickpeas
- Kidney Beans
- Lentils
- Dried Figs
- Collard Greens
- Swiss Chard
- Spinach
- Oatmeal
- Molasses
- Almonds

Zinc

Zinc is an important mineral due to the fact that it plays a major role in our immune systems and the structure of DNA. For females, the daily recommended intake is about eight and eleven if you are male. If you are a true vegan, it should be noted that the bioavailability of zinc is diminished by inhibitors in legumes, grains, and some nuts. Due to this fact, it is recommended you eat more than the recommended number so you can make sure you achieve your daily dose of zinc.

Food Examples:

- Almonds
- Sunflower Seeds
- Cashews
- Pumpkin Seeds
- Peas
- Peanuts
- Lentils
- Chickpeas
- Brown Rice
- Oatmeal
- Tofu

Iodine

For most adults, you are looking at a recommended one hundred and fifty mcg of iodine. This number will increase if you are pregnant or lactating. Iodine is very important for the production of thyroid hormones and plays a vital role in metabolism.

At this point in time, it is unclear if plant-based eaters are deficient in iodine, but it is always better to be safe than sorry! If you consume a high number of raw, cruciferous vegetables, this will be especially important as these particular foods seem to block the thyroid from absorbing iodine.

Food Examples:

- Iodized Salt
- Seaweed
- Nori
- Supplement

Protein

Ah yes, the holy nutrient everyone feels you will be lacking while on a plant-based diet. As you probably could have guessed, protein is an essential macronutrient that is in charge of several important factors in the body. You have the role of maintaining bone and muscle mass, supporting the immune system, and more.

One important factor that should be noted is that the original source of all amino acids come from plant sources. On average, people typically eat way too much protein to begin with! For adults, the daily recommended intake is .8 grams per kilogram of body weight. If you are following a balanced, plant-based diet, you should have no issues consuming the proper amount of protein!

It should be noted that plant-based eaters have trouble getting lysine. To put it simply, lysine is one essential amino acid. While it is a bit harder to come by, you can find them in many of the legumes included on the plant-based diet. Below, you will find some high protein plant-based foods for you to try out!

Food Examples:

- Almonds
- Pumpkin Seeds
- Beans
- Lentils
- Soy Milk
- Tofu
- Tempeh
- Whole Wheat Spaghetti
- Quinoa

- Seitan

Omega-3

Up to this point in your life, you have probably only gotten your omega-3 from fish. Luckily, it is possible to get these nutrients, fish-free! In fact, the essential fatty acid known as alpha-linolenic acid comes from plants and then gets converted to omega-3 within the body! This rate improves when the consumption of omega-6 is lowered so you will need to be mindful when choosing your fat sources.

Omega-3 fatty acids are important in the diet because they are linked to both brain development and heart health. The daily recommended ALA for females is about 1.1g and 1.6g for males. This number is higher for the elderly due to the fact that as we age, our bodies have a harder time converting ALA to long-chain fatty acids called DHA and EPA. Luckily, there are some easy ways to increase your omega-3 within a plant-based diet.

Food Examples:

- Walnuts
- Hemp Seeds
- Chia Seeds
- Flax Seeds

Vitamin D

To be honest, there are very few foods that contain vitamin D. This vitamin is a hormone that is produced in the kidneys to help the absorption of calcium. Luckily, we also get a majority of vitamin D from sunlight exposure which is why all people from plant-based to not should consider a supplement during colder and darker months.

Luckily, there are many plant-based foods that are now fortified with vitamin D. As a daily recommendation; adults should be getting fifteen mcg of vitamin D. The most reliable choice you should consider taking a supplement to assure you are getting the proper amount. Alongside with a supplement, you can also consume orange juice, cereals, and mushrooms.

Vitamin B12

Vitamin B12 is a hot topic among all plant-based diet. This is one of the only essential nutrients that is not made by plants nor animals. In fact, vitamin B12 is created by fungi and bacteria. Normally, this would be provided naturally on our foods, but though cleanliness and sterilization, all of the B12 is removed from the plant foods. The only reason people get B12 from animals is due to the fact that they are feeding on contaminated foods.

You may be surprised to learn that one-third of the population is low in B12; it doesn't matter if you are plant-based or not. If you are over the age of fifty, you should consider a supplement of B12 anyway. This is a vital vitamin to have because it plays an important role in red cell formation as well as the maintenance of the central nervous system.

Luckily, a B12 supplement is safe, easy, and cheap to buy! The daily recommendation of vitamin B12 for adults is about 2.4 mcg. Although this is recommended, it is impossible to overdose on the vitamin and should take a larger dose due to the fact that only a fraction of the supplement is absorbed. A daily dose should be about 250mcg or a weekly dose of 2500 mcg. On top of these supplements, you can also try nutritional yeast and fortified plant milk.

Foods to Avoid

A majority of the population is well aware of what plant-based individuals typically avoid on their diet. It should be noted that being plant-based is not necessarily vegan or vegetarian. Should you avoid meat? Absolutely. Is it the end of the world if you have some every once in a while? Absolutely not! Remember, you make choices for yourself. You know the health consequences of your actions, keep those choices in mind.

If you are new to plant-based, you may be surprised by some products that contain animal products, even when you think they are plant-friendly! I invite you to take a look at the list to follow so you can be aware of products that may be derived from animals. After all, there is power to knowledge!

Animal Foods

Yes, no duh! Being plant-based means that you should avoid animal foods as much as possible. Whether you are doing this for health purposes or for the love of animals, just be sure you try to avoid animal products as much as possible. Some of the more popular options include

Meat: Organs, Veal, Pork, Lamb, and Beef, etc.

Poultry: Duck, Goose, Turkey, Chicken, etc.

Eggs: Any Type of Egg

Dairy: Ice Cream, Butter, Cheese, Yogurt, etc.

Seafood and Fish: All Fish, Lobster, Crab, Mussels, Shrimp, etc.

Bee Products: Honey, Royal Jelly, etc.

Animal Derived Ingredients & Additives

This is where it can get a bit tricky when it comes to living a plant-based diet. One moment you are enjoying one of your favorite snacks, the next you are reading the label and realizing it has an ingredient that has been derived from an animal. Of course, we all make mistakes, but by being educated, you can avoid this mistake in the first place!

Dairy Ingredients: Whey, Lactose, Casein, etc.

Vitamin D3: Most vitamin D2 is derived from fish oil. You will also want to look out for lanolin which is found in sheep's wool. Instead, search from lichen, which is a vegan alternative.

Shellac: This ingredient is used for glazing sweet foods or can create a wax coating for fresh produce. Shellac is made from a female lac insect. Do yourself a favor and buy organic!

Isinglass: Do you love a good drink at the end of the day? You may want to check the label for isinglass. This is a gelatin-like substance that has been taken from the bladder of fish. Often times, it is used to help make both wine and beer.

Gelatin: This is an ingredient many people are aware of. Gelatin derives from the connective tissues, bones, and skins of cows and pigs. Be sure to read the label of any of your favorite snacks to avoid consuming gelatin.

Cochineal or Carmine: This ingredient is a natural dye that gives many foods their red color. This particular ingredient is made from ground cochineal scale insects. I am sorry to ruin different foods for you, but it is time you knew the truth and what is going into your body!

Sneaky Ingredients (Sometimes)

As mentioned earlier, there are foods that you will think is compliant with a plant-based diet but can sometimes contain an animal-derived ingredient. For this reason, I suggest you always be cautious and check the label on everything you eat. Better yet, try to shop as fresh as possible and avoid anything with a label altogether. If it comes straight from the ground, the chances it is compliant with a plant-based diet is incredibly high.

Worcestershire Sauce: Unfortunately, there are many varieties that contain anchovies!

Dark Chocolate: A number of dark chocolates are plant-based friendly. You will want to keep an eye out for ingredients such as milk solids, nonfat milk powder, milk fat, whey, and clarified butter. All of these ingredients are animal-derived!

Roasted Peanuts: In the production of roasted peanuts, some factories use gelatin to help the salt to stick to the peanuts.

Pasta: Some pasta will contain eggs.

French Fries: When you are eating at a restaurant, you will want to be careful when it comes down to your French fries. Often times, these are fried in animal fats.

Candy: There are a wide variety of sweets that contain gelatin. Some of the more popular versions include chewing gum, gummy bears, marshmallows, and even jelly. As you can tell, these ingredients can be very sneaky!

Becoming plant-based is going to take work. The important factor is that you are making an effort to better your health and better the world around you. If you slip up a few times, do not beat yourself up! The only thing we can do is try better next time.

As you begin to navigate the plant-based world, it will become easier and easier. Every day, we are presented with multiple food choices throughout the day. If you even comply seventy-five percent of the time, you are doing better than a mass majority of the population on their SAD diet. Just remember, if it had a face and a mother, let it be!

With all of this in mind, I want to assure that you are set up for absolute success. Next, I want you to take some time and go through all of the delicious recipes I am about to throw at you. You will find several delicious, plant-based recipes to help you get started. As you go through them, it should be noted that these recipes are meant to help get you started. Eventually, I invite you to take creative freedom and make your meals your own!

There are so many delicious foods out there for you to enjoy, all it takes is a little bit of extra effort!

Plant Based Breakfast Recipes

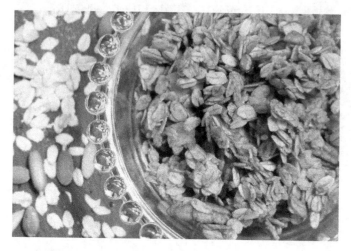

Breakfast Granola
Time: One Hour
Servings: Four

Ingredients:

- Cinnamon (.10 t.)
- Salt (.10 t.)
- Vanilla Extract (.50 t.)
- Olive Oil (2 T.)
- Maple Syrup (.33 C.)
- Chopped Nuts (1 C.)
- Old Fashioned Oats (3 C.)

Directions:

1. Granola is the perfect quick and easy breakfast choice! To begin baking your

granola, you will first need to heat your oven to 300 degrees.

2. Next, take out your favorite mixing bowl and combine the vanilla, cinnamon, salt, maple syrup, oil, chopped nuts, and the old-fashioned oats. When the task is complete, lay the mixture onto a baking sheet and get ready to bake!

3. When you are ready, place the sheet into the warmed oven for about fifty minutes. After twenty-five, you will want to stir everything together to assure even baking.

4. Finally, remove from the oven and enjoy! The granola should be stored in an airtight container for ultimate freshness.

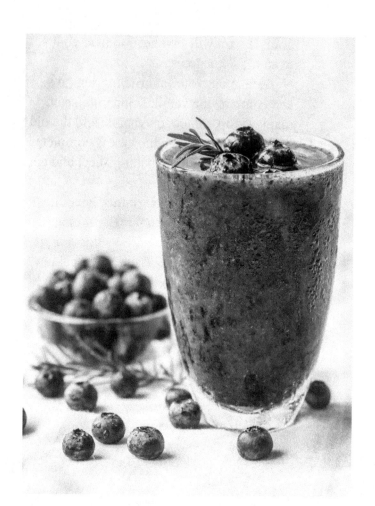

Blueberry Breakfast Smoothie
Time: Five Minutes
Servings: One

Ingredients:

- Ground Cinnamon (.25 t.)
- Unsweetened Almond Milk, Vanilla (.50 C.)
- Almond Butter (1 T.)
- Rolled Oats (.25 C.)
- Frozen Banana (1)
- Frozen Blueberries (.50 C.)

Directions:

1. Are you the type of person who is always on the go? Now, you can have a breakfast favorite in smoothie form; I introduce the blueberry muffin breakfast smoothie!
2. To create this delicious breakfast whether you are running out the door or enjoying it slowly in the morning, all you have to do is pop the ingredients from above into your blender and blend until smooth.
3. This is a great option for busy individuals as you can make this before and grab it as you go!

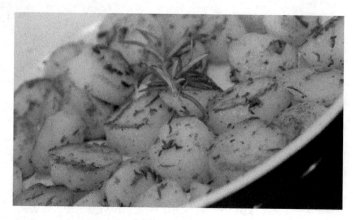

Crispy Breakfast Potatoes
Time: Forty Minutes
Servings: Two

Ingredients:

- Olive Oil (1.50 T.)
- Black Pepper (.10 t.)
- Onion Powder (.10 t.)
- Garlic Powder (.10 t.)
- Salt (.25 t.)
- Smoked Paprika (.25 t.)
- Red Potatoes (1 Lb.)

Directions:

1. For a majority of your life, you have probably heard about how terrible "carbs" are for you, and you may be shocked to see crispy breakfast potatoes in a plant-based diet book. If you look into the Starch Solution, you may be surprised to learn just

how healthy potatoes can be for you! Breakfast potatoes are delicious, packed with nutrients, and will keep your belly happy! Before you begin cooking, I suggest you scrub the potatoes down and then slice them into small cubes.

2. When this first step is complete, take out a mixing bowl and combine all of the seasonings from the list above. Once the spices are all together, gently add the potatoes in and coat evenly.

3. Once you are ready to cook, place a large saucepan on your stovetop and begin heating it over medium. When it is warm enough, add in the olive oil and potatoes. You will want to cook everything together for about eight minutes. When this time has passed, lower your heat and cook for another eight minutes.

4. The trick to making the potatoes crispy is to cook covered for the first eight minutes and then uncovered for the last eight. You will want to make sure you are stirring everything as often as you can to help create a crispy outer layer.

5. When you are happy with the outcome, remove from the heat and enjoy your breakfast!

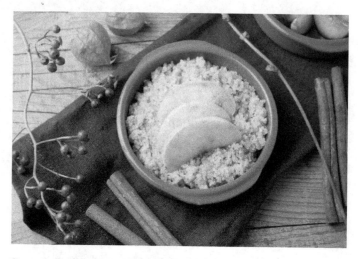

Sweet Apple Breakfast Quinoa
Time: Thirty-five Minutes
Servings: Four

Ingredients:

- Chopped Apple (1)
- Chia Seeds (1 T.)
- Raisins (2 T.)
- Stevia (1 Packet)
- Cinnamon (.25 t.)
- Water (.25 C.)
- Almond Milk, Vanilla (.25 C.)
- Dry Quinoa (.25 C.)

Directions:

1. This Apple and Cinnamon Quinoa dish is one of my favorite breakfast foods. The sweetness of the apple and cinnamon truly

compliment one another without feeling too sweet for the morning time. This is a perfect option if you have a few moments to truly enjoy breakfast. If not, you can always make it ahead of time and enjoy it later on!

2. To start this breakfast recipe, you will want to get out a saucepan and place it over a high heat. When this is in place, put your water, quinoa, and milk in. I would stir everything together just to make them combine better. You will want to bring everything to a boil before you reduce the heat and put the cover over the top.

3. After about five minutes of simmering this mixture, you can remove the top and add in the chia seeds, chopped apple, raisins, stevia, and cinnamon. Once this is complete, continue to cook everything together until the liquid is all gone. Generally, this can take between ten and twelve minutes, depending on your oven!

4. Finally, remove the pan from the top of the stove, decorate with more cinnamon and apple slices, and enjoy this sweet breakfast treat!

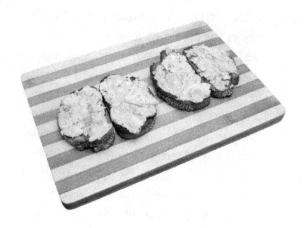

Avocado Toast
Time: Twenty Minutes
Servings: Six

Ingredients:

- Whole Wheat Bread (6 Slices)
- Black Pepper (.10 t.)
- Red Pepper Flakes (.25 t.)
- Olive Oil (1 t.)
- Salt (.10 t.)
- Balsamic Vinegar (1 t.)
- Avocado (1)

Directions:

1. Fun Fact: Avocado contained twice as much potassium when compared to a banana. With all of the fiber and oleic acid to help our digestive tract and heart health, perhaps the millennials were onto

something with this avocado toast obsession!

2. If you need a fun and easy way to add some healthy fats into your diet, avocado toast is the way to go. To begin, take out the favorite mixing bowl of yours and combine all of the ingredients from the list above. Obviously, leave the toast out at this point. Once everything is mixed together well, you will want to place the spiced avocado into a food processor and blend until smooth.

3. Finally, slather the avocado onto toasted bread and breakfast is ready! For extra flavor, I enjoy sprinkling more red pepper flakes over the top. This is your breakfast; make sure you enjoy it to the fullest and season however your heart pleases! There are many, incredible ways to enjoy avocado. I invite you to try several different varieties to find your favorite.

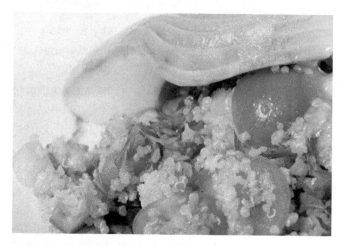

Quinoa and Black Bean Bowl
Time: Ten Minutes
Servings: One

Ingredients:

- Chopped Fresh Cilantro (2 T.)
- Pico de Gallo (3 T.)
- Diced Avocado (1)
- Lime Juice (1 T.)
- Hummus (.25 C.)
- Cooked Quinoa (.50 C.)
- Black Beans (.75 C.)

Directions:

1. This bowl is the perfect lunch with its blends of delicious flavors and nutrients. This one dish is packed with twenty grams

of protein! On top of that, it is also plant-based friendly and will be ready within ten minutes! Before you begin assembling your bowl, you will want to make sure you cook your quinoa according to the directions on its package first.

2. When this first step is complete, get out a mixing bowl and carefully combine the quinoa with the black bean. When this is complete, squeeze your lime over the top and gently stir in your hummus until you reach your desired consistency.

3. Finally, top the bowl off with fresh cilantro, Pico de Gallo, and diced avocado! For extra flavor, you can also try adding in half a package of taco seasoning. I also enjoy adding in some of my favorite vegetables for more flavor. I added corn and tomatoes, but you can put in whatever you enjoy!

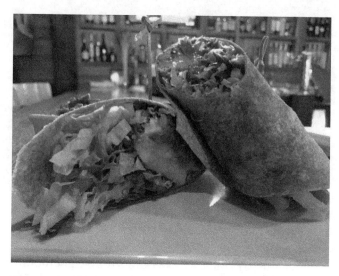

Hummus Wrap
Time: Fifteen Minutes
Servings: Four

Ingredients:

- Shredded Lettuce (1 C.)
- Diced Avocado (2 T.)
- Diced Tomatoes (1 T.)
- Black Beans (2 T.)
- Corn (2 T.)
- Southwestern Hummus (4 T.)
- Whole Wheat Wraps (4)

Directions:

1. If you are looking for an easy lunch to whip together when you are low on time but is still healthy and plant-based, this hummus

wrap will be perfect. Between the black beans, avocado, and diced tomatoes, your mouth will be filled to the brim with flavor! Be sure to find whole wheat wraps to help keep this recipe as healthy as possible.

2. Once you have gathered your ingredients, you will want to lay out the wraps and carefully and evenly spread the hummus across the top. When this is complete, you can begin to assemble the wrap with the shredded lettuce, tomatoes, black beans, corn, and the avocado.

3. Carefully wrap up your lunch and enjoy!

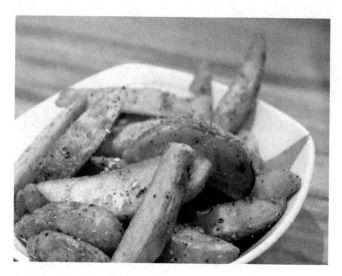

Baked Potato Wedge Fries
Time: Sixty Minutes
Servings: Four

Ingredients:

- Olive Oil (3 T.)
- Pepper (.50 t.)
- Paprika (1 t.)
- Garlic Powder (1 t.)
- Flour (2 T.)
- Onion Powder (1 t.)
- Salt (.50 t.)
- Russet Potatoes (4)

Directions:

1. We have all been there; sitting at your desk or on the couch and suddenly, the fry

craving hits you! It happens to the best of us! Now, there is a healthy option so you can get your fry fixing! Luckily, this recipe is delicious and easy. Before you begin setting up your fries, you will want to heat your oven to 450 degrees. As the oven warms up, you can prepare a bake plate by drizzling it with the olive oil and then place it to the side.

2. Before you begin preparing the potatoes, you will want to make sure you scrub them down well, and then pat the potatoes dry with a paper towel. When this step is complete, carefully slice the potatoes in half, lengthwise, and then into quarters. By the end of this, the potatoes should be in thick wedges.

3. Next, get your mixing bowl out and combine all of the dry ingredients from the list above. When this is complete, pop the potatoes into the bowl and mix around to coat the potatoes evenly. When this is complete, spread the wedges out onto your baking sheet evenly.

4. When you are ready, pop the sheet into the oven for around twenty minutes. After twenty minutes, you will want to flip the potatoes to their other side to make sure you cook them through. The total time of baking your potato wedges will be about

forty minutes. After this time, remove from the oven and allow to cool down.

5. Finally, enjoy these potato wedges alone or with another delicious plant-based meal!

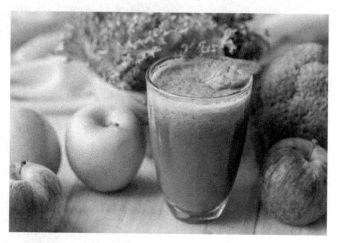

Green Detox Smoothie
Time: Five Minutes
Servings: Four

Ingredients:

- Ice (as needed)
- Water (.50 C.)
- Almond Milk (.50 C.)
- Chopped Pineapples (1 C.)
- Chia Seeds (3 T.)
- Bananas (2)
- Kale (3 C.)

Directions:

1. There will be moments that you slack on your diet. This isn't necessarily your fault but sometimes life just gets in the way, and we don't make the best of choices. If this sounds like you, this smoothie will do your body some good. It is simple to create and chalked full of the nutrients that your body is craving. Say goodbye to feeling sluggish and hello to feeling fresh and free.
2. To create this recipe, all you have to do is place everything from above into your blender and blend on high until smooth. It should be noted that the level of ice can be changed depending on your desired consistency. For a thicker smoothie, add more ice. If you like it to be thinner, you can add more water or milk depending on what you want!
3. Finally, pour the smoothie into your favorite glass and enjoy!

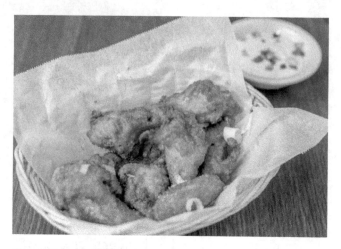

Cauliflower Wings
Time: Thirty-five Minutes
Servings: Four

Ingredients:

- Nutritional Yeast (2 T.)
- Curry Powder (1 t.)
- Garlic Powder (1 t.)
- Chickpea Flour (.75 C.)
- Onion Powder (1 t.)
- Almond Milk, Non-sweetened (1 C.)
- Buffalo Sauce (.75 Bottle)
- Cauliflower (1 Head)

Directions:

1. As you go more plant-based, wings may be one food that you "miss" from your SAD diet. Luckily, these cauliflower wings hit pretty close to home! They are crunchy,

chewy, full of flavor and the best part, healthy! It should be noted that you can make these with any of your favorite sauces! I chose buffalo sauce for this recipe because I love spice! You can try making these any way you desire, just be sure to check the label to assure there are no hidden animal-derived ingredients! When you are ready to cook, heat the oven to 450 degrees.

2. As the oven warms up, you can prepare the head of cauliflower by chopping it up into florets. When this is done, set it to the side and prepare the batter by combining the spices, flour, and nutritional yeast. Next, add in the flour and carefully stir everything together. Once the batter is created, you can dip the cauliflower into the mixture and space evenly onto a baking sheet.

3. Once every piece of cauliflower has been coated, pop the sheet into the oven for about twenty minutes. By the end of this time, the cauliflower should be nice and crispy. If it isn't, you will want to leave it in for a bit longer.

4. Once the cauliflower is crispy, remove from oven and place back into a mixing bowl. At this point, you will want to douse the wings with your favorite sauce. For this particular recipe, I chose my favorite buffalo sauce for an extra kick! When the cauliflower is

well coated, place back into the oven for another twenty minutes or until the outside becomes crispy. Remove from the oven, allow the cauliflower wings to cool and then enjoy!

Dinner Recipes

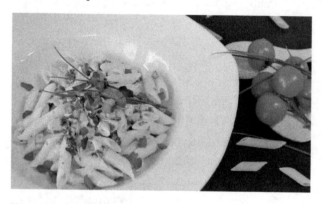

Tomato Basil Pasta
Time: Twenty Minutes
Servings: Five

Ingredients:

- Spinach (3 C.)
- Salt (.50 t.)
- Fresh Basil Leaves (.25 C.)
- Vegan Cream Cheese (.50 C.)
- Fire Roasted Tomatoes (1 Can)
- Whole Wheat Penne (16 Oz.)

Directions:

1. For a quick and healthy dinner, this is a wonderful plant-based option! This meal is fantastic because it is yummy for the tummy and doesn't have a load of complicated ingredients. Just six ingredients and you will have dinner on the table within twenty minutes! To start, simply cook your whole wheat penne depending on the directions located on the package.
2. As the pasta cooks, you can blend the rest of the ingredients together in your blender to create a sauce for the pasta. Feel free to season the sauce to your own desires. There is plenty of room for experimenting when it comes to cooking!
3. Finally, you will want to place the cooked pasta into a large skillet and carefully pour the homemade sauce over the top. Once everything is in place, turn the oven on a medium heat and sauté the pasta for a few minutes. At this point, add in the basil leaves and cook until the leaves become wilted. For extra flavor, try adding more vegetables to your dish! I added chopped tomatoes and fresh cilantro over the top for some added flavor.

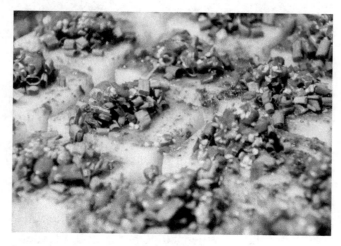

Baked Tofu
Time: Forty Minutes
Servings: Four

Ingredients:

- Cornstarch (1 T.)
- Water (2 T.)
- Minced Garlic (1)
- Grated Ginger (1 t.)
- Sesame Oil (1 t.)
- Dry Sherry (2 T.)
- Rice Vinegar (2 T.)
- Soy Sauce (.33 C.)
- Brown Sugar (3 T.)
- Water (.25 C.)
- Black Pepper (.25 t.)
- Cornstarch (1 T.)
- Olive Oil (1 T.)

- Soy Sauce (1 T.)
- Diced Extra-firm Tofu (14 Oz.)

Directions:

1. If you have never had/made tofu before, it can be a bit tricky. I put this recipe in here to push your cooking skills. While it does take a small amount of extra effort, it will be worth it when you have a healthy dinner waiting for you on the table! When you are ready, gather all of your ingredients and then we can begin!

2. First off, heat the oven to 400 degrees and prepare a baking sheet. Personally, I like to line mine with parchment paper, but you can grease with oil if you would like.

3. Next, place the tofu into a bowl and cover with one tablespoon of the soy sauce along with the olive oil, salt, and the pepper. Be sure to toss the tofu well to ensure even coating. This is vital to spread the flavor through your whole meal.

4. Once the third step is complete, you will want to place the tofu onto the baking sheet. Be sure that you evenly space the tofu, so the pieces cook at an even pace. Go ahead and cook the tofu for about thirty minutes. Halfway, be sure to turn the tofu on the other side, so all sides become nice and crispy.

5. As the tofu cooks in the oven, you can make the sauce. You will do this by mixing the ginger, garlic, sesame oil, sherry, rice vinegar, soy sauce, brown sugar, and water into a saucepan. Now, bring the saucepan to a simmer and cook sauce for ten minutes. You should expect the liquid to reduce by about a third.

6. When this is complete, take another small bowl and carefully mix together the cornstarch and water. Once done, add into the sauce and stir well. By the end, the sauce should be nice and thick!

7. Once the tofu is nice and crispy, remove from oven and place into the saucepan. You will want to stir everything well to make sure the tofu is well coated. For a full meal, try serving over brown rice or with some of your favorite vegetables. For extra flavor, you can also add scallions and top with sesame seeds. Serve and enjoy your hard work!

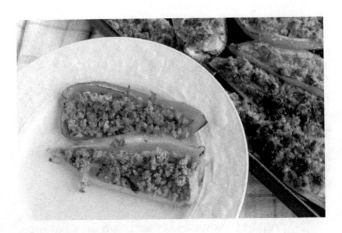

Stuffed Peppers
Time: Thirty-five Minutes
Servings: Four

Ingredients:

- Dried Oregano (1 t.)
- Red Wine Vinegar (1 t.)
- Garlic (1 Clove)
- Black Olives (2 T.)
- Pine Nuts (2 T.)
- Quartered Cherry Tomatoes (1 C.)
- Low-Sodium Chickpeas (1 C.)
- Cooked Quinoa (1 C.)
- Red (Yellow or Green) Bell Peppers (2)

Directions:

1. Talk about a nutrient-filled dinner, say hello to one of your new favorite dishes! These stuffed red bell peppers provide filling fiber along with antioxidants, vitamin A and

vitamin C! This meal is easy to prepare and can be stored in the fridge for several days if you need a quick and easy meal! When you are ready to start cooking, go ahead and bring your oven to 350 degrees.

2. As the oven warms itself, take your red bell peppers and cut them down the center. At this point, you will want to remove the stems because let's be honest, nobody wants to eat that part! Once these are prepared, you can set them up on a baking sheet.

3. Now, get out that mixing bowl and stir together the rest of the ingredients from the list above. When this is finished, carefully spoon the mixture into the red bell pepper halves.

4. Next, you are going to pop the baking dish into the oven for twenty-five minutes. At the end of this time, the peppers should be nice and soft. For extra flavor, try sprinkling parsley over the peppers and serve warm.

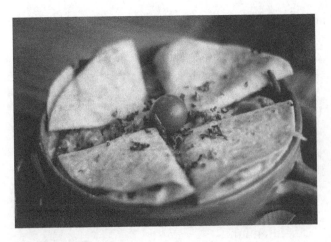

Crunchy Wrap
Time: Forty-five Minutes
Servings: Four

Ingredients:

- Whole Wheat Tortillas (4)
- Tostada (4)
- Taco Seasoning (1 t.)
- Dried Green Chiles (1 Can)
- Water (.50 C.)
- Cashews (1 C.)
- Salsa (.50 C.)
- Chipotle Peppers (2)
- Taco Seasoning (2 T.)
- Firm Tofu (16 Oz.)
- Olive Oil (3 T.)
- Optional: Black Beans, Cilantro, Lettuce, Tomatoes, Avocado, Salsa, Tortilla Chips

Directions:

1. As you can probably already tell, this delicious meal is the healthy take on your favorite handheld tortilla pocket from Taco Bell! It is loaded with delicious vegetables, tofu, and vegan CHEESE? You are probably asking yourself how in the world is this even possible? Honestly, I would rather show you than tell! It is going to take multiple steps so be sure to pay special attention.

2. First, we are going to prepare the tofu. You will be completing this task by heating a large pan over a high heat. As it warms up, you will want to take your tofu and crumble it apart with your hands. When this is complete, add in the salsa, salt, and the taco seasoning. Allow this to sit for ten minutes without touching anything! If you need to, add oil on the bottom of the pan to prevent anything from sticking. In the end, the tofu will be browned and pretty crunchy! Perfect, go ahead and set that to the side.

3. Next, it is time to make the cashew queso! This can be done by taking a blender and mixing the cashews, water, a tablespoon of the taco seasoning, and the can of diced green chilis. If you don't like spice, add fewer chilis. Blend until everything is

perfectly smooth and then set the cheese to the side.

4. Now, it is time to assemble the crunchy wrap! Begin by laying your tortilla on the counter. The layers go, tofu, crunch part (I used a tostada) and then any other extras that your heart desires! You can use lettuce, tomatoes, salsa, avocado, black beans, corn; literally whatever you enjoy! Once everything is in place, carefully fold the tortilla toward the center and then place to the side.

5. When you are ready to cook your meal, place the seam side down onto a skillet and cook over medium heat. Usually, it will take a few minutes to brown on either side. You will want to cook through until the exterior is firm and browned; otherwise, it will just fall apart.

6. Finally, remove from heat and enjoy!

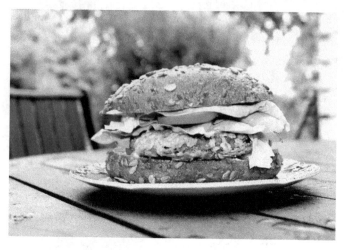

Black Bean Burgers
Time: One Hour
Servings: Eight

Ingredients:

- Dry Breadcrumbs (3 T.)
- Ground Flax Seeds (1 T.)
- Pepper (.25 t.)
- Chili Powder (.50 t.)
- Ground Cumin (.50 t.)
- Salt (.50 t.)
- Dried Oregano (.50 t.)
- Black Beans (1 Can)
- Jalapeno (2 T.)
- Chopped Onion (.25 C.)
- Fresh Ginger (1)
- Garlic (2)
- Old Fashioned Oats (.50 C.)

- Walnuts (.50 C.)

Directions:

1. Yes, you still get to enjoy burgers while following a plant-based diet! These black bean-based burgers are easy to make and delicious. To start off, you will want to get your food processor out. Once you have it set up and ready, add in the jalapenos, onion, ginger, garlic, oats, and walnuts. Next, pulse everything for ten seconds.

2. Once the first ingredients are blended, you can add in the flaxseed, pepper, salt, chili powder, oregano, cumin, cilantro, and beans. When everything is in place, process for five seconds intervals or until the beans are mostly broken down. You will want beans to stay whole for some extra flavor.

3. Now, carefully scrape this mixture out of the processor and place in a bowl. Once this is complete, place in the fridge and chill for fifteen minutes or so. After this time has passed, add in the breadcrumbs and use your hands to combine everything together.

4. With the mixture made, begin to shape patties; you should be able to make seven or eight patties. When you are ready, pop the patties onto a skillet over medium heat and cook for about five minutes on either side. By the end, the burgers should be a nice golden-brown color.

5. Remove the burgers from the pan, place on a whole wheat bun, and go to town with plant-based toppings! Whether you use lettuce, tomato, ketchup, mustard; make it a fun family activity!

Chapter Four: Common Misconceptions and How to Overcome Them

When you first begin a plant-based diet, you should expect a lot of doubters in your life. There are many people who don't understand this way of life because they simply do not know or understand the facts. Within this chapter, we will be going over some of the common misconceptions that come with the plant-based territory. By the end, you will be able to answer just about any of the common questions that will be thrown at you.

Myth # 1: A Plant-based Diet is Not Healthy

People have a hard time accepting the concepts that they do not understand. I want you to take a moment and think about your current diet. More than likely, your diet is just like everyone else's. Eating plant-based will bring you numerous advantages over your typical SAD diet. As you learned in the second chapter, there are several benefits of starting a plant-based diet including reduced risk of cancer, lower rates of obesity, weight loss and more. You very well know that on a plant-based diet, you will be able to get all of the nutrients you need and more.

Myth # 2: Going Plant-based Means I am Vegetarian or Vegan

The notion that you will be a vegetarian or vegan on a plant-based diet is an absolute myth. Overall, the goal is to have less meat and in smaller portions. If you have fish every once in a while, or a piece of meat, it will not be the end of the world. As long as you are putting forth the effort to evolve your diet around vegetables, fruits, and unprocessed foods, you will be doing incredible things for your health. If you are just starting out, remember to start small and cut it out slowly.

Myth # 3: Eating Plant-based is Too Expensive

There is a terrible misconception that eating healthy means that it is going to be expensive. The good news is that there is a way to eat healthy while following a budget. In the chapter to follow, we will go over this a bit more in depth. For now, it should be noted that many of the foods you will be eating include whole grains, legumes, and beans. These ingredients all cost less than fish and meat! The key is to buy fruits and vegetables that are in season. When you start eating less meat, you will have more money for your grocery budget!

Myth # 4: Eating Plant-based is Boring

In the chapter from above, we slightly touched some of the delicious foods you will be able to eat on a plant-based diet. If you are following this diet properly, at no point should you feel deprived. In fact, there is a very wide variety of foods you will be eating that are filled with nutrients and extremely healthy. Next time you are at the grocery store, take a few extra moments to browse the produce aisle. You will be surprised all the different legumes, fruits and vegetables you can try out! On top of this, you can also explore new styles of cooking and ethnic foods. I highly suggest you try foods and new recipes; there is always room to grow.

Myth # 5: I Need Meat for Protein on a Plant-based Diet

This is one of the top questions you will get while following a plant-based diet. Your friends will suddenly become a nutritionist and worry you are not getting enough protein how that you are no longer eating meat. The truth is, instead of eating animals for their protein, you are going directly to the source! As you very well know at this point green vegetables, beans, and nuts are all excellent sources of the protein you need on a daily basis.

Myth # 6: I Need Milk for Strong Bones

There is often a misconception that we need milk to grow strong bones. The truth is, we need calcium and vitamin D in order to grow strong bones. Most of the calcium within our bodies are found in our bones. When we lose too much calcium in our diet, it could potentially lead to osteoporosis later in life. As you know from the earlier chapter, there are plenty of ways to boost your calcium intake on a plant-based diet. Be sure you are consuming the proper foods such as fortified plant milk, beans, dried figs, or sweet potato to keep your daily calcium intake up.

Myth # 7: Going Plant-based is Too Hard

This is where I will disagree the most with the doubters. When you think about it, making any changes is extremely difficult. There are many individuals who start diets and fail, and that is because they don't believe enough in themselves. This is why your WHY is so important. Why are you choosing to follow a plant-based diet? Is it for health purposes? Is it to lose weight? No matter what your why is, that reason is reason enough to overcome any difficult times you will come across with a plant-based diet. True, change can be hard, but as you practice more, your lifestyle will become much easier!

Chapter Five: Tips and Tricks

Before we send you on your way to your new healthy lifestyle, there are a few important tips and tricks for you to learn and keep up your sleeve. In the beginning, it always seems easy to begin a new diet. You have this new found motivation and energy to change your life. But, what happens when that energy burns out in a few weeks? By knowing some tips and tricks about the plant-based diet, these will keep you going when times get rough!

Getting Started on a Plant-based Diet

1. Find Your Motivation
   Truly, I cannot express the importance of this enough! If you are here in this book, there was probably something drastic that made you want to make a major change. This reason is your why and what you should set your goals around. Whether you are looking for mental clarity, more energy, or helping a disease, always try to remember why you are starting this lifestyle in the first place. For bonus points, write down your why on a sheet of paper so that you can look at it when you need added motivation.
2. Remember to Eat

As mentioned earlier, a plant-based diet is very filling when you are consuming whole foods. It will be important that you remember to eat more than you are used to. Luckily on a plant-based diet, you can say goodbye to counting calories. Now, you can fill up on salad, fruit, quinoa, beans, and even baked potatoes to your heart's content! The whole point of this diet is to live off the good food, and over time, the body adjusts to the volume of food. After a while, you will learn to rely on your satiety cues and natural hunger.

3. Prepare Food

As you start a plant-based diet, I encourage you to take a stroll through your kitchen. In the beginning, you will begin to recognize the foods that may not be as beneficial to you as a whole food. I suggest you toss these foods or give them away, so you keep yourself out of temptations reach. Instead, fill your fridge and pantry with healthy foods such as beans, rice, and potatoes! This way when you get cravings for unhealthy foods, there won't be any in your house!

4. Take it Gentle

Switching over to a plant-based diet does not need to happen overnight! Instead, I suggest taking a gentler approach and slowly switch your diet to become more plant-based. If you make sudden changes, you could potentially feel restricted and ultimately cheat yourself out of your amazing diet. An example would be to use avocado instead of butter! While it is a change, it will take some time to get used to. As you increase the healthy plant-based ingredients in your life, you will slowly eliminate the bad stuff.

5. One Meal at a Time
There are no rules saying that being plant-based needs to be a now or never type of deal. Instead, try switching one meal at a time to be more plant-based. One of the easier meals, I have found, is breakfast! Instead of your normal milk and cereal, give oatmeal with your favorite fruit a try! There is also delicious avocado toast or breakfast potatoes! I highly suggest trying some of the recipes provided in this book to help you get started! Slowly, you can switch all of your meals to being plant-based, and soon it won't even be a second thought.

6. Find Good People
I mentioned earlier that many people close to you will doubt your lifestyle choice, but there are also many likeminded people out there in the world that are going through the same changes as you. Typically, it is easier

to go through changes when you have company to share your struggles and successes with. It is a fantastic idea to form a support group so you can reach out for help and inspire others. I suggest checking out internet forums or even Facebook groups for you to connect with. Just remember that you are never alone on this journey!

7. Keep it Fun

   Switching to a plant-based diet is not meant to be a form of torture. I hope that eventually, you learn to enjoy your food choices and perhaps even look forward to it. Luckily with modern technology, you have recipes at your fingertips. There are always new foods to try and recipes to give a shot. A good way to keep your diet fun is to have an adventurous side. The next time you visit the grocery store, I challenge you to choose out a fruit or vegetable that you have never heard of before. When you have made your selection, use the internet to find ideas on how to cook this item. You may be surprised at what you learn about food and about yourself!

8. Commit

   As you begin the plant-based diet, the best thing you can do is make the commitment to yourself. There are a number of reasons people begin the plant-based diet. Why are you here? Why do you feel a plant-based diet can change your life? At the end of the day, it does not matter what anyone else thinks. If you want to make this commitment to yourself, you make this commitment! It is time to take your health into your own hands. You are the only one who can make health decisions for yourself, make sure those decisions are the best ones possible. You owe yourself that much.

Plant-based on a Budget

One major excuse individuals use not to eat healthily is that they feel eating healthy can be too expensive. The trick here is to make smart choices. There are plenty of ways to strip the diet down to the basics; whole foods can actually be easily affordable for just about anyone! All you need is some knowledge about whole foods, and you will be able to fit all of your nutrients into your budget with ease!

1. Stay Home!
   This seems like a given but eating at home instead of going out to a restaurant can save you a lot of money whether you follow a plant-based diet or not! Instead of dining out several times a week, eat out for an occasional treat! If you are constantly on the move and rely on fast food, begin to

prepare snacks in advance. This way, you will have full control over your meals and what goes into them. Also, by staying home, this will give you a fantastic chance to work on those cooking skills!

2. Choose Whole Foods

   While this may seem like a given, whole foods are going to be some of the cheapest staples you can buy! Luckily, the whole foods are going to offer the most essential nutrients as well! Some of the more popular, budget-friendly foods include brown rice, oats, potatoes, carrots, leafy greens, frozen vegetables, apples, oranges, other fruits in season, and all of the beans and lentils!

3. Think Big

   Not literally, but when you buy food in bulk, you can get much more bang for your buck! When you are at the grocery store, look for the big packages or family packs. Typically, these will provide better value compared to smaller bags or containers. In this case, you will want to pay special attention to the unit price located on the price tag; this number will tell you the cost per pound. By following this rule, you can choose the cheapest option.

4. Keep it Simple, Stupid

   If you are just starting the plant-based diet, there is no reason to get crazy and wild in the kitchen! Just because you are switching your diet, this does not mean that you need to become a crazy, skilled chef. Keeping your meals simple does not mean that they are going to be boring. As you can tell from the recipes earlier in this book, recipes can be easy and delicious at the same time. Often times when you use too many ingredients, this makes it tough on the pallet and your digestion tract. Do yourself a favor and start small. As you get better with this lifestyle, that is when you can experiment a bit more with your meals.

5. Buy in Season
   This is vital when it comes to shopping for a plant-based diet on a budget. The good news is that food that is grown in season is cheaper and tastes much better. In the winter, keep an eye out for citrus fruits and root vegetables. In the summer, you can keep your eyes out for nectarines and watermelon. Do yourself a favor and visit your local farmers market to get the freshest produce possible. You may be surprised to learn the wide variety of food that is made available to you!

6. Frozen
   Lastly, frozen fruits and vegetables. These items are typically cheaper and can be very convenient. Frozen fruits and vegetables are typically picked once they are ripe and then

frozen right away; this meaning that the foods will maintain their nutrition. This is a fantastic idea, especially in the winter when fresh produce may be limited on variety and quality. Just remember to read the label of ingredients so you can avoid any added butter, sauce, or seasoning.

Meal Planning 101

While there are several hurdles you will be facing as you start a plant-based diet, one of the more popular issues is planning your meals! In the beginning, it is exciting to try out new recipes and be on point with your nutrition. Eventually, many people begin to slip up and then give up their goals of eating healthier altogether. Luckily, it doesn't have to be as complicated as people make it out to be! Instead, you can arm yourself with these meal planning tips and tricks to help you get through when you come across a tough hurdle.

The first question you may have is why should you plan your meals? As you begin a plant-based diet, you may find it to be more difficult compared to planning meals on a SAD diet. Now, you will be slightly more limited on the foods you can have during your meals. This is why you need to educate yourself on how to properly plan your plant-based meals! Planning is vital so that when you are short on time, there is less decision making. With meal prep, you won't overthink your meals and will be prepared at any given moment.

Meal prepping is also vital to help you stick with your healthy habits. By planning ahead, you will have a lower grocery bill and be able to eat your daily nutritional needs without thinking about it on a daily basis. This is especially helpful if you are looking to lose weight! At the end of the day, you know what will work best for you. If meal prepping will help keep you accountable, it is absolutely worth the extra effort.

Before you begin the meal prepping, I suggest starting a food journal. As you cook different meals, you can start at the beginning and keep track of the foods you enjoy and the ones you don't like so much. This way, you can save time and effort when you are trying to plan meals. This can also help you stay organized with your ingredients. In the beginning, you should keep everything simple. This way, they can be batched easily and repeated in future meals.

Choosing Foods to Prep

One of the most important factors of meal prepping on a plant-based diet is the foods you are going to include on your meal plan! I want to stress that this is meant to be fun and enjoyable. Below, you will find some of my favorite tips and tricks to keep meal prep delicious and easy.

- Look for pre-cut or frozen foods; it will make your life ten times easier. Yes, it is more expensive, but you pay for convivence!

- It is okay to adjust! As you will find out, most recipes are not one taste fits all. If you feel a certain recipe is rather bland, add your own seasonings! There are no rules stating you need to stick to the recipe or else! Express your inner chef and season to your heart's desire.

- Make a list. Seriously. As you meal prep, make your grocery list as you go along. This will help you stay focused and organized when you get to the grocery store. Making a list is also a fantastic way to avoid buying foods you really shouldn't.

- Making a list is also a wonderful way to save money. This way, you will know exactly what you have at home, and nothing will go to waste. Often times, this can be a big issue with fresh produce; it doesn't have as long as a shelf-life compared to processed foods.

- Remember to add variety to your meals. Being plant-based does not mean that your meals need to be boring. There are many flavors and spices for you to try out! Experimenting is one of the best parts of a plant-based diet. You just never know what is going to spark your taste buds!

- Stick with foods you are going to enjoy. If you don't like Brussel Sprouts, don't buy them! Are they healthy? Yes. Does that mean you need to force them down your throat? No! There are plenty of options out there, keep your taste buds happy!
- Stock your kitchen with staples. There are some wonderful choices such as potatoes, lentils, quinoa, millet, beans, and rice. These are fantastic to have as you can build multiple meals around the staples. Remember that these are going to be the centerpieces of your meals from now on. Choose one and build around that ingredient and you can never go wrong with your plant-based diet.

If you are ready to commit to the lifestyle of a plant-based diet, there is no better time than the present! You have all of the information you need to help you get started; all you need to do is apply your new found knowledge of this lifestyle. Is it going to be difficult? At first, absolutely. Change can be incredibly hard, especially if you have eaten the same way your whole life. All you need to remember is that you don't have to make the changes overnight; in fact, you are encouraged to start slow! Soon enough, you will begin experiencing the health benefits, and you will wonder why you didn't start earlier. All you need to do now is believe in yourself and make that dive!

Conclusion

Before you leave, I want to congratulate you on making this healthy choice for yourself. Changing your lifestyle is not going to be easy, but it is going to be worth it! Whether you are doing this for health reasons, weight loss purposes, for the love of the animals, or saving the environment, I hope that you are going to put this book down and feel prepared for your new journey.

As you continue down the path of your plant-based life, feel free to come back to the chapters of this book any time you have a question. I encourage you to try new foods, push your cooking skills to the limit, and always remember why you started. I wish you the best of luck on your new, healthy journey. Live well and enjoy life.